NOT MY FAULT TO LOVE YOU

Gary a Young Man who frolic with girls since his youthful age fell in love with Lily a beautiful girl who came from a very poor back ground. After being together in love for some years Gary ask Lily hand in marriage, unfortunately pregnancy occur, before she think whether she should accept Gary hand in marriage. but she couldn't even believe her self, she requested for money from her boyfriend for test whether the pregnancy is positive.

In the hospital doctor Dan tested her and prove to her that she's pregnant. on her way home are Heart was fill with joy to accept to Marry him. she expected to found him at home suddenly she didn't seen him. she ask her neighbour, she told her that he just walkout with is a visitors to the childless hotel, Lily reply thanks and left. Lily think what to prepare for her fiance likeness she prevail, to prepare him is favourite meal she known that his fiance like eating pepper soup rice with goat meat she prepare the meal as fast as possible before his fiance arrived.

His fiance was very happy more than her, he had ring in bucket. at arrival at home he received a hug that he did not seen nor feel in is entire lifetime after that Lily bring him is favourite meal as they repast the meal she told him everything. Gary was full of unamountable love and he propose to her say"marry me and be my love forever" with no Denel she accept. they became one blood that was a great day for them.

At night Lily was dreaming how she is discussing with is mother-in-law about her pregnancy, what the child sex will be. they were guesting that the child will be a girl {say by is mother} her mother-in-law say that it will be a boy so that I may have second son/grandson but in their village the honour grand son more than her mother.

when Lily awoke she was amazing because she did not seen her mother-in-law before In her dream. she call his fiance

"when will we go to the village?"

Gary answer "meaning"

"I mean to visit my mother in-law"

"is they any problems"

she say "no but I only want to see her so that she may bless my child"

"we will go tomorrow morning".

when morning came they all prepare to the village. on their way going Gary saw her friend {Merab} since from his secondary school they were surprise of themselves, then chatting take place.

she asked about Lily "is she your sis"

Gary replies "yes a sister in Christ

"how"

he reply "my wife".

she was excited and asked"you also pregnanted her? and she turn to Lily congratulation for marring my friend I wish you successful birth through

she reply "Amen".

 the relax in the hotel called {De choice} after all she left.

Gary and Lily want to the village, they get into compound they saw their mother peeling cassava and they join her. after some minute she call her house maid to peel the cassava they get inside the house she was jubilant of seeing her daughter in-law pregnant.

she entertained them with joke, some minute later are daughter in-law was walking around the compound, then she use that opportunity and call his son for some interviews about the girl pregnancy, behaviour, character whether she is a real African woman who knew how to take care of the family.

he reply"she has over come all {meaning} she is excellent in all. his mother was confirm and the return to the sitting room. Lily return to the sitting room for permission to join Abigail to peel the cassava she was surprised of seeing her husband, she join him and the baby in her womb dance too. the house was fill with love her mother-in-law pray for the baby In her womb. at evening Gary asked her mother to shown him all his father properties documents, she bring him the documents box he open the box saw is father pic, because is father died young he cry, every body console him to forget about his death father he Stamps the files and return it back to is mother. in evening the left to their home in town.

three month later Lily feel very painful and restive she was taken to the hospital there she delivers a bouncing baby boy when Gary heard the goodnews   that her wife have deliver a baby boy he feel very happy to the point he could not describe nor narrate is happiness. then he rush to the hospital with some baby clothes and thing. in the hospital he call her mother to come and stay with her daughter in-law, when her mother came he left to buy some of the baby thing on his way returning to the hospital he had and accident and dies his was off head. the hold story turn to bad news.

the man was buried with   grieve and every body cry and mourn him for two months he was a very good man handsome , kind and have self control.

but in eight days after the baby was born and the father was dead the name after is father Gavin.

after Gavin naming ceremony Lily her mother was back from the hospital and live with her mother-in-law so that baby will be treated to the conduct of Annang people. she stay there with her mother-in-law and help her on some house choice also to farm but her mother-in-law always ask her to stop stressing her self it is not up to one month when she give birth she keeps no response.

one day she was had the farm weeding, her mother-in-law was discussing with her friends about Lily that she didn't knew she is a African woman who can work very hard tidy up the environment. on the farm she had finish weeding resting under palm   tree a man came with bag she greeted, he answer, came close to her consoling her about his dead spouse. after a minute he also narrate how a widow should forget about spouse that the man had gone. Lily was sock about the man word thinking that the man is up to something he ended his word by asking Lily to have sex with him she reply"I will never allowed any man test my spouse private hood"he keep a bag full of money to accept for the sex she rejected it.

then he hold her with force damage her clothe to rape her she put are finger into he eyes he fall down, she ran away. at home she didn't found her mother-in-law she changed up are dress before Cecilia her mother-in-law came back, she narrate everything she reacted by calling the police the man was arrested before Cecilia send Lily back to her home town. the man was jail three years the case ended.

At the city, it was around 8pm when Gavin and his mother went to bed, they slept comfortable at 1am doit. Gavin heard a sound heating the door he ran to his mother Lily, Lily was in a very deep sleep Gavin try to wake her. unfortunately Gavin heard a sound of foot step walking in the house he ran to the next room to hind, immediately he ran to next room the thieves enter the room and Robbed her mother. her mother was beating, he heard how they treated her mother   he took by the back door an ran out of the house for help. when Morning came Gavin was no where to be find he got missing, her mother   search for him all over the town centre but he couldn't find him. she went to the police station and make a report about the missing boy, the police make some investigation but the couldn't find him nor located him.

she find it difficult to located his son, so he spent close to a week trying to find him. He asked whoever care to give him attention if the had found Gavin but no one knew Gavin by that name.

worse still, he hardly associated with people. Even if he met him he wouldn't have recognised him because by this time Gavin had completely emaciated. he was haggard and dirty. Gavin was at Etinan. he was at Etinan junction doing conducting work for drivers he was very smart till the driver where looking for him. one day he meet one fair woman, who he was thinking she is a passenger the woman approach him and talk to him one to one as a mother the associated with her. Gavin accept to be her house boy.

At Merab house, Merab had a son named Paul, Paul was aged nine while Gavin was eight years old. Gavin live there for two months and became the favourite of the family. he was very loving, peaceful, kind and smart.

On the other hand, Paul Merab son was rude, jealous, disrespectful and proud. this make Merab loved him dearly but Paul was always jealous of Gavin. any time Merab warned him of the consequences of his lifestyle he would frown and cry complaining that they only cared for Gavin. Paul wanted everything he saw buy hardly would he share it with his friends and relatives.

One day, his best friend, Udo went on holidays to his uncle in Lagos city. he came back with lots of goodies assorted colours, toy and snacks. on arrival from Lagos Udo rushed to Paul's house with everything he brought back. he couldn't wait to Change his clothes against his parent's advice. quickly, he rushed to meet his friends whom he had missed.

On seeing Udo with the item Paul rushed o garb the bag from him. he didn't care to greet his friend. his whole attention was on the bag his friend his holding. Udo knew he loved such things and was excited to see him admire everything in the bag

Udo asked him if Gavin but didn't get any reply so, he went inside and met Gavin in the studio drawing. they exchanged pleasantries and went together to the children's sitting room where Paul was playing with the toys while eating some snacks from the bag.

He appeared not to notice anybody, Gavin picked one of the toys but Paul snatched it from him immediately. Udo wanted to struggle with him but was quick to understand his behaviour. Udo wanted to get back to work to avoid scene but Gavin wouldn't let him go. he had to pick some toys and snack for Udo, thought Paul objected.

At evening Udo told his friend he would like to go back home with the toys so he could show them to his parent before giving them out. Paul was disappointed at such news, "that can't be done " he said "if you didn't want to give them to me, why then did you bring them here? I thought these thing are mine, you promised to bring me gift from your uncle's house. you won't go with the again",he mumbled. "please let me go back now, you can see it is becoming late and my father wouldn't be happy if I spend minute more here or do you want the to punish me", Udo pleaded. this didn't go down well with his friend who kicked everything in about of anger.

Fortunately, Paul mother arrived at that moment and embarrassed at her child's attitude. they apologized immediately on behalf of the family. they also packed the items for the boy who had started crying.

Udo was escorted back home by his friend's mother   since he said his parent would be mad at him for flouting thier order. he couldn't have gone back alone since it was too late. when Paul mother got back home, he was given some stroke of cane for being greedy, ungrateful and rude to his friend.

he was deprived from the suya meat and fruit drink his mother bought for him and Gavin on her way back. if there was anything painful to him it was the suya was his favourite. he asked Gavin to sneak some meat for him as he often did at other times but the boy was tired of unrepentant attitude. his lifestyle was becoming unbearable. at least, that punishment could serve as a deterrent to him. Gavin the house boy knew the punishment was well deserved.

Paul woke up the next day Angier than he was before going to bed. he felt nobody loves him even his mother. this thought provoked more hatred toward Gavin. when Gavin greeted him in the morning, he bluntly refused   to respond but this did not bother Gavin since he knew Paul hardly forgave. he thought that with time he will get over it but his wasn't to be as Gavin was planning to hurt him in revenge. they where in the same school. Gavin was in   primary five while Paul was in J.S.S1 of the secondary arm of the school.

Normally, Merab dropped them in the school before going to work while they go back on thier own at the close of school. Paul was warned never to leave Gavin behind.

However, on the fateful day Paul decided to leave Gavin to pay him back home for the incident of the previous night. He took Keke (tricycle) back home knowing well Gavin had no money with him to pay back home even if he was he is of age to that.

Gavin look for him everywhere in the school but Paul had gone home much earlier. he didn't understand why Paul could go home without him. the boy though of how he could get home alone and thus made him to cry.

In addition, Gavin was hungry and needed to get home in no time to eat his lunch. he would have called her house mother but he was afraid she will punish Paul when they got home. he decided to turn his misfortune to an adventure if sort. he decided to trek home with some of the older students of the school.

At a point, he was all alone because none of the student lived along his street. as he was walking he started humming some poems he learnt in school so as to wade off feat especially when. he got to lonely path.

It was at the point that he caught a picture of a a very lovely cat. Gavin was attracted to it. he couldn't help but drew closer to have a full view of the artistic piece. he had always loved animal especially butterflies with glittering eyes and this particular car had semblance. the cat had finer colour.

The cat refused to run away even when Gavin. was moving very deeply to it. Gavin wouldn't go back, he moved on with confidence and the cat began to jump around that place. Gavin sang a song he had learnt from his grandmother for the lovely animal and the cat appeared happier drawing closer to his new friend. the cat opened its mouth and Gavin could see some glittering objects inside the animal mouths. Gavin tried to pick up the cat but it wouldn't follow him. the amazing cat vomited the shiny objects and a voice directed him to pick them.

Initially, Gavin hesitated because her mother have always warned him never to take anything which doesn't belong to him. he contemplated how he would explain his actions to his Merab when he got home. he didn't understand such act of benevolent from a reptile.

The voice told him this came as a result of his uncommon kindness and humility. the cat was able to convince him that these rare gifts is from God.

Finally, he obliged and picked the beautiful stones. he wouldn't know what the objects were because he had not seen them before. anyway, he was attracted to thier charm and considered them as toys. Gavin didn't know how well to thank the animal for that show of kindness. immediately, the cat ran back into the bush.

He was over- excited to be rewarded that way and he had forgotten he was hungry. the hunger had to vanish because if joy. strolling home with the objects in hand, he saw his house mother car driving toward him. Merab was shocked to find him unaccompanied on a lonely path. refusing to ask questions, he went out and picked him into the car. he was more surprised to find some gold with Gavin. the woman almost screamed if not he had always learnt to control her temperament. "where did you get those items, do you know what they are, in short what were you doing there?" Gavin didn't know which to answer Frist but tried to start with the Frist. "it was a cat who gave them to me and I think they are toys", he said with confidence."I will give to Paul, some to our friend, Udo and kept some for myself", he continued. his house mother refused to talk again as he was becoming confused of the scenario. she only told herself he needed to get home, to Paul so he could get fact from him.

as she got home, Paul started crying thinking her mother would punished him from abandoning Gavin at school.

Gavin patiently explained everything that happened to Merab who gave thanks to God for rewarding Gavin with such expensive gifts. he told Gavin those were gem- Stone's they weren't toys as the lad had thought

This was a lesson to Paul who was always means, greedy and jealous. he regretted his lifestyle and decided to new leaf. he was happy to learn from Gavin to be nice to others. but this called for celebration said by Merab, Gavin and Paul was directed by Merab to dress up for shopping, they went to a hotel called (DE CHOICE) they jubilant, enjoy, cheer up but in the order way it was a boarding for Gavin about are mother. which make him to feel sick.

Lily is a Doctor, she was transferred to hospital near Abak road (emergency hospital) she was there over five months ago. Gavin house mother did not notice that Gavin had   malaria fever. Gavin try to prevent it but the sickness developed fever he could not walk nor eat, he was taken to general Hospital the rejected the patients.   everybody was worried without explanation why Gavin did took them he is sick. Now the search for a hospital and they discovered the emergency hospital near Abak roads

At arrival, In the hospital he was admitted to bed for proper treatment he was handle by nurse Oliver. on the next day Merab was In the hospital, Lily Gavin mother approach her siad "hi" Merab did not even have time for her, she was nervously to without attend. within two seconds Merab live the reception office to   Gavin ward, Gavin was feeling better but still cold. on the day Gavin arrival at the hospital one patient was death. so the hospital manager put in order that all the doctor most check on the patients, has morning duty the was a roster. it was Lily duty to check the patients in every ward, as she was on the process, Passing through Gavin ward she heard a sound mummy Merab reply, "am not calling you" said by Gavin he stream "Mummy" Lily turn back and look forward for the caller. he couldn't recognised him, he stream all over before Lily, lily perambulate to him "mummy, me" repeatedly Lily didn't notice any thing, all she was thinking he had a high blood pressure. because Gavin was emaciated, Lily want to test him he hold her hand, called "mother me Gavin" her mother look towards him called "Gavin!"he replied "Mum" she crow triumphantly jump up and down exulting. had she was shouting all the doctor's and nurses gather the were shock of such voice, asked why are you shouting, she replied"is complicated rejoice with me I had found my missing child". she order for drinks, every body drink and jubilant with her. immediately she rush to the manager office for perceptible about her son. the manager asked her to narrated what happened, after the summary of the brief statement her requested was granted. Gavin Instantaneously out of the hospital the settle the hospital pilled and when to Merab house.

At Merab house Gavin was felling excited of seen are missing mother he called his friends for celebration why his mother and Merab where discussing in the parlour. Udo and Paul was with Gavin. Gavin stood them that he is leaving with his mother, there where all Playing Ludo enjoying snacks bought by Gavin. in the order hand Paul was sad because Gavin was like a brother to him. "but we'll, there is nothing I can do" Paul heart dictation. when it was 4pm sun was going down, Gavin prep his belongings and follow his mother the left to thier home town. Merab and Paul missed him a lot.

one years later Gavin as grow to level of starting secondary school, he was very brilliant and been intelligence. at his fifteen years old the boy was in SSS 1 {senior secondary school} her mother rented a house for him near the school compound so that he may focus on his education many of his friends fall in friending girls and having girl friends. but nobody knew why he appeared to secular and hate the idea of wanting to play with girls he was very afraid of girls because girls like distraction. Gavin give no attention to them, Gavin knew that keeping the girls away from him is a very   difficult thing, in all he was the most handsome boy and black in complexion jolly decent incase of looking back twice to him.

the girl had the right to disturb him, he had been fund of communicating with one of them the reason why he exchanging word with this girl is she is brilliant not having stupid idea like them. He separate him self and kept a cross bay for them.

Aileen one of his classmates planning to communicate with him she wrote a letter to him by James his friend the next day James bring the letter to him he read the letter he say to James"I am very disappointed in you he give the letter back to him without written any thing In it, Aileen was feel with hatred.

every body in the class wonder without explanation why Gavin did not involve him self in love affair. in SSS 2 Gavin saw and alien getting inside the class room he ask"who is she? Peter replied"she a new student Gavin said"okay because she is not with her school uniform" he demand to known her Peter was surrogate why Gavin want to know the girl name he reply"I don't know" it was 2:00pm school closed.

At home he was feel romantic love about the girl he heart beat with love evendo in his dream, he dream about the girl he didn't even care to read his book and assignment,   when he woke up he remembers all that happens to him yesterday he said"what is coming after me , I my insane? {rhetorical questions} he gear up to school, at school no aid constant to teacher nor sitting in class the only thing he did is go to girl section watching her, he could not even go close to her nor ask questions. returning back home he wrote a letter. early in the morning, on Monday he toke the letter to his friend Peter to surreptitiously bring it to her. at arrival had her site Peter greeted her she answered he ask"please Aunty what is your name? she "Linda", Peter said "my friend Gavin ask me to bring this to you "she answer "thank" she receive the letter reading take place after she had finish reading reluctantly reply"I had no choice than to accept I have such a feeling" she return the letter back to Peter with are response Peter return back to him. Gavin was relished with love not even care how to speak with her that day because of relishness

on Tuesday Gavin goes straight to her not even drop his bag, he didn't not found her in her site he wait for her to return when she came back she didn't even respond or regarded him immediately she turn to aloof. Gavin was amazing of her attitude he was embarrassed he return home with grieve, he wept very painfully in the house. when Peter went to return his not to him he open the door and get inside he was him crying he ask"Whatsapp? he reply "Linda rejected me" he was   shock of him crying for a girl he console him to be a man he say it repeatedly he was Abid with the word and stop crying.

At class he was in a reflective mood he was quiet aid reflective boy. Linda narrate story to James, James was unbelievable Mary confirm with evidence that is true. Linda expose the secret concisely then James was relished and blackmail the news to all classes and sections in concisely ways some of the girl who he didn't not accept to be their boyfriends collide Gavin he is pretender

when Gavin heard how James and Linda embarrass him it full with conciliation because of God.
The relationship of Gavin and Linda was tense emotional feeling involved of hatred.
END

IT'S PAYS TO BE GOOD

For All Human Beings In The World.

A long time ago in Obio Imo village, there was a poor boy called Edet, he was living with his poor Mother who was a widow, they had no place to lived, but they usually slept at the church Surender. they were poor still the extent thy would entered the bush in searching of kernel, the used this money to fried Akara, they would hawk around the whole village still the points villagers gave then name "Akara mio " it was the course of this that Edet and his mother lived thier village to the neighbouring village because the feel so embarrassed due to the name given to them by the villagers.

One night Edet had a dream of selling plates, he then woke up and told his mother's, his mother was so pleased but she was worried about were to took the money for the starting up of the business. Edet and his mother struggle to searched some kernels and thier church also contributed some amount of money for them in order to used and feed themselves. But Edet saved the money, latter he took it to the market and bought some plates and started trading.

Edet started selling plates and some house hold utensils he earned a lot from the business. However he had a nice thought about building of small Mud house for himself. he met his old friend Mr. Udoita who was a professional in building Construction. He told Mr. Udoita all his planned, he was very lucky that Udoita accepted and reflected for him bamboo trees and they both join hand together and construct it with the bamboo trees and mud.

Edet packed his belongings to his new apartments, he went to Urua-ibaba and rent small repository for his goods.

Two years later Edet   married to Miss Eno, a citizen of Usung Ubiom village, Eno lived with her uncle because her biological parents we're death. Eno had two sister named Ukut and Emem, she was fair in complexion, a damsel and a hard working lady, although she was not educated but she had a sound thinking vacuity. Edet was attracted with all these characters of Eno and he sought and won her hand in marriage, he went and meet Eno family and her uncle for pride price, after paying the bride price, they gathered all the villagers for traditional marriage, in the ceremony people ate and testify Elder and chairman were server with kola nuts, bitter Kola and palm wine. the Village head Mr. Inuen Ekpo blessed the couple, the chairman gave a closing remarks and dismissed the visitors, Edet and his wife returned home happily.

Some months after the traditional marriage, Eno conceived and gave birth to a young Baby girl. Edet was so excited till the point that he assembled all the family members for child namiling ceremony, he named the child Eno-Mfon and changed the mother's name from Eno to Inem.

Inem was able managed her marital home and she do not want to depend on her husband, then she got herself involved in petty trading she followed her husband to Urua Ibaba and bought some food items like Garri, Cray fish etc. and sold in small quantities to the people.

One day as Edet was returning back from the market, he met a group of robbers and they were shooting sporadically Edet tried with all his might to escaped but unfortunately he was caught and they size   from him his bicycle, his goods and the sum of ten thousand Naira, they beat him mercilessly and he was left empty handed without any thing apart from the remaining twenty thousand naira which was hidden in his inner wear the cried unruly and went home anxiously.

Edet through the help of his wife and the remaining lucre, he tried and make up again, he realised that going to the market to sell his goods would caused him a great failure, due to the anxiety that was in him, he went and rends a ware house where his goods were sold and stored.

Edet became a popular trader and was known by many foreign traders due to the state of slave trade, at this point Inem gave birth Again to two more children's, this time the babies were male children, (Akpan and Udo), they both grew up to the cogent of getting to final year in secondary school and thier father was employed in the same school as a labourer for additional lucre. Mr. Edet earned a lucre that he planned for a stone building bricks, due to insufficient water, the children in order to assist thier parent, in house construction project the went to the neighbouring houses and collected some bicycles and some rubbers which they used it to far distances so   that they could found stream and fetch water, they usually went to Ndem stream in order to fetch, one day in the dry season, the stream was dried and the could not found any water. the children were worried about such a situation, on thier way home they met an old man and they all greeted; good morning sir, the old man replied morning children, "is there any problem?" ask by the old man. "No" the children replied, and the old man said "why are you worried" Akpan said in a low tone "it is because of lack of water in the stream," the old man said "don't worry my children, we had so many stream around us, like Umoh stream" and the man directed them to the stream, they all fetched, thanks the man and went home, they thought of seeing such a faithful man again.

After some years when the building was completed. Edet impregnated his wife and she delivered a bouncing baby boy Joe. at this time Akpan and Udo had wrote thier WAEC and looked for a job to do in order to earned a living, they both make decision to go for Apprentice, Udo was send to Aba to learn how to produced, sew and sell shoes and bag. Udo was very skillful in shoes productions, bags and others, he made more lucre from his job, he planned of making another thing that would make him to earn lucre, he discuss with his elder brother and his sister, they both make contributions that he should get involved in road and building construction he rejected the suggestion. he told his siblings that he would like to sold clothes, napkins, baby pampas, creams, bath etc. the suggestion was a accepted by his siblings, he moved further and told his parents. his parents, we're so excited for seeing such a idea. they gave him word of advice and prayed for him, he then bud his parent and sibling farewell.

while Udo was going on with his occupation he got a lot of wealth, he bought a plot of land, be built a house he fulfilled of making oil mill.

Joe was now a big boy who had passed through primary education he was agile in nature, he always went to different churches for counseling, he was strenuous in order to fought his brothers he always do things which is bombshell, he swindle his parent and had a lack Luster attitude towards their family issue.

on one   fateful day Udo got to his shops, he open and sweep, suddenly a Whiteman greeted using a saccharine voice, Udo was impressed he told him bring some material like bath soaps, towel, handkerchief   etc. the price was given all was set by transfer, Udo again had   more lucre from the man to improve his business. this make Udo business to boom he fulfilled building borehole water in his compound, Joe was ill-fated he tries to fought his brother, people always advice him about his bad attitude and his siblings did the same yet Joe did not listen, he became a nocturnal, and a very greed friend to his brothers.

Joe went to the best secondary school in the village, he always use false word to collect money from his parent. Akpan his elder brother was now a professional in electrical work, he always teaches some of his follow colleague. his master like him more than others. he was so assiduous in his work, he was usually send by his master to go and withdraw some money from the bank. his master do this in order to test his faithfulness and contempt.

Akpan was freed from the work his master make a great celebration to him and announced that he is the best servant he ever had. his parent and relative could no longer hold back themselves. they surged forward to embrace and hug him. it was a joyous day in thier family, Akpan was well known as an electrician, he had many servant and won so much contract, he usually went to the market and bought climbing robe,and took to his shop and sold.

As time goes on, thing became difficult for Akpan, and it was the will of God because he wanted him to work in his vineyard and Fisher of Soul for christ. Akpan on his way to shop, he approached a mad man, the mad man prophesied unto him on the term "go and be a Fisher of Soul for christ " Akpan was shock and he had no choice than to deviate from electrician to a preacher. as he was a strong member in the church and one of the youth executive leader, he was appointed by the church councils that he should be one of the new seminarian. Akpan was excited. he prayed to God to grant him favoured in order to succeed in life, because he always had a depression about success. the following day, he went to the white men Christian church seminary and collected a form, he was told to filled it. when he finished filling the form, he returned it to the directors in charge for the form it was taken to America.

Two weeks latter Akpan was giving a letter to start as a seminarian in the church. he was assiduous in his studies, as they were still in the junior seminary all the seminarian were examined before the cross over to the senior seminary, some of them failed and they were sacked but Akpan was more intellectual that he took the third position and was promoted with some of his colleagues to the senior seminary.

Akpan was   brilliant in such a way that he always helps to make editaubles in the seminary and he also helps to resolute conflict between his colleagues and also among the lecturers, by this points in time he was more popular and regarded as one of the best seminarian.

when Akpan was still in the church seminary his brother Joe had finished his secondary education and his father gave him some hug amount of money to used and started a business, he took some some of the money and enjoyed with harlot and later bought a camera, he used this camera to make a hoax he always collected money from the people without returning the photograph and ran away to a place called "plaza" and stay there, whenever he went there he would took some of his brother climbing- rope for selling but the money will not be refunded. Akpan his brother dislike is attitude and tried to correct him from such art but he could listen and form a animosity to him.

Each time he ran away with people money his brother or father will handle for him. and did not want to change from it, but he tried to get improved in his arrogant life.

After a year Akpan was promoted to the post of an evangelist, so it was time for them to took the final examination before promoted to a vigar, and due to how the student were competing in their last exams the lecturers were impressed and they made a   law that the first three people's would be taken to America for more training but due to some jealousy by the senior pastors who were leaders at that time argue that it was not done for them, how could little seminarians be taken to America said the senior pastors, Akpan who was one of   the first three people's to came out of the exam was unable to went to America.

Further more, it was time for Akpan to be ordained he must be married. Akpan has a poor boy whom came from a poor family had no choice than to looked for a lady whom will pleaded with him, he met a fairly damsel whom he sought her hand in marriage, and she accepted gave a condition that if only Akpan would accompany her to her church and become a member that she would wed him. but in return Akpan told her that he was about to be ordained as a pastor in this church and he is unable to lived and pleaded with her to accept it, but she rejected and Akpan move on for another person.

One fateful day, Akpan woke up and prayed to God for a faithful, lovely and hardworking woman, he was looking for a government worker, as he finished with is prayer he met one of his colleague who was med and discussed the issued, when the colleague wife heard this, she went and told them that there is one lady whom she knew that has all this characteristic of a lady that Akpan wanted. so Akpan was directed to the lady and she met the lady and discussed the issued and the lady accepted to marry him. after Akpan marriage ceremony he was ordained as a pastor.

He encounters a lot of troubles during his ministry work. Joe his brother was great threats to his ministry work, Joe fell in love to a little girl from Akpan Esit-Ikot Iba but the lady's father warned him to stay clear from the girl and he refused, on the mood he got the girl pregnant. when it was time for delivery the girl was unable. unfortunately the girl gave birth to a baby boy and died.

Joe was very sad and stay without food for three days thinking of his present situations. at time goes on he went and met his father and his brother Akpan by this time Udo his brother was death due to I'll health. Joe went with his family members to the house of his late wife, as they were there they were ordered to seat. they greeted, no one replied they perceptible discern to them harse and he was ordered to med the corpse by paying the bride price and a lot of money was spent by his father and brother, but Joe himself has no money to support himself. since the situation was worst in such a way they can not handle Edet carried some plot of his land and sell to Akpan (temporary) in order to rescue Joe. Akpan because of love took he took the money that he want to use and goes to Lagos and start business and gave to his father and Edet took the money and paid the bride price for Joe late wife. latter Edet and his son joined together and buried the girl for Joe

some years latter Edet was sick and Akpan tried all means to to served his life but all was invalid and Edet gave up at the age of seventy nine. his sons, wife and only daughter mourn and need no consolation.

Following the tradition of the land, it was time for Edet to be buried and the family members gathered and planed for the burial. Joe has joined a bad gram and planned on how to claim his father's properties, Joe causes disaster every where in the village and tried with his might to annihilate his brother, he went to the white men Christian church and condemned his brother so that his brother will be sacked but the elders of the church did some investigation and knew that Akpan is innocent about that blackmailed said by Joe.

Joe without the feared of God went to the land that was sold by his father to Akpan in order to rescue him and have some palm fruits from the land and said to his cabinet that the land was not sold by his father, that Akpan just want to claim the land, that if it is so, let him brought the agreement book, since there was no agreement book, Joe was able to claims the land, when that was not enough for Joe, he moved further to fought his brother's wife and removed her tooth, chest his brother with machete and condemn his brother's motor cycle.

When it was time for God to retaliate him and gave him the reward of his work. a planning committee was held against his father's burial. Joe went to postpone his father burial without any reason, and it was remaining only one week before the burial. the people rejected his ordered, he then entered thier midst and scatter every things, he told the people to lived the compound. suddenly the family head commanded him to sit down and siad "young boy why are you behavioristic like this? can's you have respect for your elder's? Joe was so annoyed and angry with the word he surged forward and slapped the family head. thus make they youths to be so annoyed and provoked, Joe, after he had slapped the family head, he wanted to escaped and he was reprehended and castigated by the youths, they were angry till the points the used machete on him and the he was latter hand over to the police.

Joe was unable to attain the burial due to his bad behaviour. after Edet burial, Akpan was promoted to the rank of Bishop. because of blessings he received from his father and how he was patient, loyal, faithful and we'll behaved.

Following their church doctrine he was send to America because Bishop don't served in their country. Akpan was excited and he knew that God has answered his prayer about success and before he moved to the airport in order to take his flight he quickly remember the advice of his father which says "it pays to be good".

END

THE MAGIC BEAN

There was once a boy named Uko, who had a little sister, Aky. They had a horse as a pet. The horse was trained to hear sounds. It could run long races without getting tired.
The horse also fought vigorously. It was an extra ordinary white horse with wings to fly high up the sky. It was very
beautiful, robust and clean. Uko promised never to sell it because it was a piece of admiration to the whole community.
Aky was barely two years but she used to follow Uko to school. She could recite a few rhymes and sang songs she learnt in class. One day, when her brother was preparing to go
to school, Aky told him she wasn't going to school. He thought it a joke because Aky has always loved school. Uko
only realized it when he wanted to dress her for school and she
objected. He tried to convince her with some promises that
their mother who had left for the market at dawn will buy her
many gifts.
His brother tried to persuade her to no avail little, did he
know that Aky wasn't feeling well. He thought she may have
wanted to stay with their cousins to play. So, he left for school
without her.
On getting back home after school, he expected to see his
-sister playing with other children outside but didn't. He went straight to the room and found her writhing in pains. She was crying and there was no one to attend to her.
He shouted to draw people's attention and as expected, they rushed in to help him. One of their neighbours offered to pick their mother from the market which was not far from the house. The poor woman rushed home to meet her sick daughter crying.
A herbalist was called to administer treatment. He did what he knew but Aky wasn't getting better rather her health was deteriorating. The whole family wept bitterly asking for help from relations because there was no money to take her to the   health center. Uko's mother suggested he should sell their lovely horse in order to save her dying daughter and he obliged.
On his way to the market, he met an old man who wanted to buy the horse, many others had wished to buy it but almost all the villagers were poor like
Uko's family. It was very difficult to make
money in their village since
everybody practised subsistent agriculture. The women only traded by barter, they
exchanged goods for other goods they needed. Uko hoped to sell the horse to any stranger who happened to go to the market that day. The old man bargained the price with him and Uko expected to collect the money so he could rush home to attend to Aky. To his surprise the old man handed him a bean.
Initially, he rejected it but the old man was able to convince him to collect it. The man told him the bean could give him fortunes in life when planted and he believed him. After all, old men don't tell lies.
In the euphoria, Uko rushed back home with the bean in his hand. He considered the bean a precious gem and handled it with care. He thought of many things he would do when the bean grows as the old man had promised. To his greatest dismay, his mother scolded him harshly on hearing his cock and bull story. The neighbours didn't believe him either. They thought he must have hidden the horse somewhere since he loved it dearly. Some thought he may have kept back the money, "children of these days you can't trust them", they said shrugging off their shoulders. The mother was completely disorganised because the horse was their only hope. To worsen

things, their father had not yet returned from the king's errand. He had left for the land of Ovie two days earlier. Everybody in the family felt sad that Uko couldn't help his ailing sister while others believed that he had been swindled. Since nobody believed him he went alone in search of the old fraudster but the old man was faster than he could imagine. He knew Uko might get back to look for him, so he ran away with the horse as quickly as possible. Mr. Akpan was shocked to see a crowd in his compound, he asked for explanations from the sympathizers. They drew his attention to his daughter who was rolling on the floor he almost slumped but was helped by the people.

When told about the sale of the horse and the story behind it, Mr. Akpan was very furious, he called Uko who was no way to be found. He roared like a lion asking everyone he met for Uko. As he approached the road, Uko was running towards the house. Instead of waiting for him to arrive the man rather ran towards him. He caught his son, beat, kicked and even bit him. People tried to reScue Uko from his hand to no avail. The more he beat him the more confused he was, trying to figure out what his fault was and why nobody believed him. "Daddy, please, don't kill me allow me plant the magic bean

and you will know the truth, I can't deceive you", he explained amidst tears. "Shut up, you thief, I'm afraid you are not my blood because I have never stolen a pin in my life, how much did you sell the horse, if you don't produce the money now, I will bury you alive", his father threatened.

Uko's mother had to abandon her ailing daughter to rescue Uko having known her husband's temperament, but her effort only provoked the man themore. She tried to persuade him to leave him so that they could take their daughter for treatment before she gives up. At that, Mr. Akpan disowned Uko, went home and threw away all his personal effects.

A caring relative who worked as a security guard in the Health Center happened to come back from work to witness the pathetic scene. He rushed the poor girl to the clinic. Meanwhile, the father refused to follow them to the clinic. At the health center, Aky was only given First Aid since her situation was too bad to be treated in that facility. She was referred to the General Hospital for proper attention. Surprisingly, no money was demanded by the health

workers as expected because the child was under the age of five and the state government had approved free medical care for children below this age bracket. They didn't have to pay for treatment both at the Health Centre and the General Hospital. Aky was placed on admission at the General hospital and they spent about a week there. Mr. Akpan never visited his wife and daughter for once

during this period.They only lived on the benevolence of

nurses, other patients and some charitable organisations   who visited the hospital during the period.

Unfortunately too, Uko was

thrown out of the village by his father. His father sneaked him out of the village at midnight when nobody could notice it.

Uko was lying down on their veranda when his father took him away even without his personal effects.

He made sure he was abandoned where he would never be able to trace his way back home. His father warned him strongly never to go back home since he has disowned him. The hard-hearted man threatened to kill him if he ever dares to go near the village. Uko cried his heart out begging him for mercy even if he had sinned. This seemed to provoke his father the more. "Any day I see you again near my village I will kill you, live on the street where you can steal as much as you like, I hate thieves and would never accept a thief for a son", he roared. Uko wept sore throughout the cold night wondering what may have happened to his only sister. He wondered how his poor mother would feel when she eventually comes back to discover that her only son has been

sent away. Will she go back home with Aky or will she live a

barren woman if Aky happens to die? These bothered him the

more when he remembered that he was his mother's pet and confidant.

His father has always been very harsh even with his wives, so Mrs. Akpan took solace in her children. Some said he was a

wicked man but he never believed it until he lashed out this evil act on him.

"Oh, could it be that since he has many children from his other wives my father doesn't like me? How do I cope without a family"? Uko kept asking himself. He never knew there were

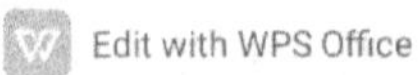

children living on the street in their community. He only read about street children in books.
For days Uko cried without consolation, he found a home in the town hall which was always open.
There were other children living there but he refused to associate with them.
These children were wild, violent and disgusting. They were very dirty, bathing once in a long while.
Uko was quite a stranger among them. In the day time the boys would go around town packing rubbish for people who offered them a token which they used in feeding.
The female folks went round town with whoever cared to pick them. They were very wayward and unkempt. People said they were witches and wizards. It was generally believed that the killed their relatives which prompted the community to expel them. He wondered why
fate would bring him to live with such caliber of people. This made him cry the more.
One day, as he was crying, a street boy tapped on his back. As he turned, he was appalled by the kind of figure that greeted him. "Leave me alone, I'm not one of you. I want to go home and meet my
mother and sister", Uko screamed.
"There is no point crying over spilled milk, we are now your friends, here we live like a family, as you can see we are happy and if you join us you will be happy too. No amount of tears will fix those things for you again if they so loved you why did they throw you out or you think we don't know your parents don't want you anymore", said the haggard looking boy.
Uko was resolute and would not join them, after all, he wasn't of their stock. The poor boy knew he was only there because his mother wasn't at home. He knew one day he would go back home to the warm embrace of his mother. "But how on earth could a father be so heartless and what crime did he commit", he pondered.
That was how Uko came to live on the street. He became dirty and haggard. Young boys of his age and older ones would even beat him up. They threw stones and sticks on him even
without provocation. Oh, how they despised him without cause.
The street boys hated him because he refused to join them in committing crime and he didn't accept gifts from them though he was always very hungry. They also thought he slighted them by not playing with them.
Uko only accepted things from a good Samaritan woman, Mrs. Sam who lived near the village hall. The woman noticed he was different from other children living there. So one day, she asked him what he did to have warranted this kind of treatment and he told her everything about the magic bean'. He even showed it to her. She had wanted to take him back to his mother but Uko didn't know the name of his village. He only knew his father's name. She only consoled him that one day, his mother would find him.
Mrs. Sam pitied Uko after hearing his story. She also
watched him closely and knew he was only a victim of circumstance. Others condemned him including her husband who warned her to beware of street children because they were all criminals. She often gave him toiletries and food
items. The woman even bought him a few clothes and would have taken him home if not that her husband opposed the idea
strongly. Uko used to call her Mummy and this made him remember his real mother with nostalgia. Sometimes, he
doubted if he will ever meet his mum and loving sister again, the questions went on and on bothering him.
On their return from the hospital, Aky and her mother learnt in dismay that Uko had been thrown out during the
period of their absence. Mrs. Ben wept bitterly for her son who has been harshly punished. She reported her husband's action to the family head who tried to advise Mr. Ben on the negative effect of his action on their son.
Mr. Ben denied sending his son away. He explained that Uko ran away because he wasn't ready to live with him again.
He also said Uko ran away so that he could enjoy the money he stole with his other accomplices and would come back the
moment the money is exhausted. When they asked if his son
has ever stolen before Mr. Ben answered that he had been pretending all along. He said that Uko has been influenced by bad friends in school.

The case was reported to the village head who summoned him immediately. Mr. Ben was asked to bring back the boy or face the full wrath of the law. This was the decision of the village council. For fear of being banished and his properties seized, Mr. Ben had no choice than searched for his son. He found it difficult to locate the place he dropped his son, so he spent close to a week trying to find him. He asked whoever cared to give him attention if they had found Uko but no one knew Uko by that name.

Worse still, he hardly associated with people. Even if he met the poor boy he wouldn't have recognized him because by this time Uko had completely emaciated. He was also haggard and dirty.

However, one day when Uko was bathing in front of the village square, he saw his father speaking with one elderly man, Immediately, Uko ran inside and hid himself to avoid being seen by him. He thought he was coming back to kill him as he had threatened, so he refused to go out for the next two days.

He would have died of hunger if his foster mother didn't visit him with food. Afraid that the woman might ask him to follow his father, Uko refused to confide in her even when she asked why he did not come out to get food from her as usual.

After a fruitless effort of ten days, Mr. Ben went back to the village to ask for leniency from the village council. He was given a period of grace to find him but was directed to report the case to the nearby police station. He knew what that meant and would not dare report himself to the police ratherhe chose to request for more hands from the youth leader who obliged in the interest of the missing boy, Uko.

One day, as Uko was selling water on the main road Uko caught sight of an object which bewildered him greatly. He couldn't believe his eyes, so he needed to go closer, behold it was his horse. See my horse, he exclaimed, this attracted other boys to the scene. The rider couldn't recognize Uko may be he would have run away. So he stopped when Uko begged to mount the horse for N20.

As soon as he climbed the horse and the horse noticed him andjumped in ecstasy. "This is my horse, old man you deceived me and ran away with my horse, everybody please comne", he shouted.

The man tried to argue with Uko but since the horse could recognize him it was certain Uko was saying the truth.

"Everybody come oh, I have found my missing horse, please save me from this fraudulent old man", he screamed with all his strength.

By this time all the street boys were alerted and they rushed down to defend one of their own who was sub-changed by a hardened criminal.

They were furious that the criminal was walking freely on the street while the victim was still serving his harsh punishment. They had heard the story before though not directly from Uko. But for the intervention of some security operatives, the old man would have been lynched to death, they wanted him to pay for his actions, after all everybody thought all the street children are devils, while others were saints.

Atleast they wanted to prove a point to the world that some of them who are on the streets are victims of injustice and unfairness. Uko's foster mother was also there, she explained to the people what the man's action caused the poor boy and they were shocked and sad. They regretted calling all street children devils.

The old man, Uko and the horse were taken to the police station. The horse refused to follow the old man as directed by the security operative. Rather it was Uko who rode it.
At the station, they were asked to give their statement, the old man refused to talk until he was beaten by the police man on duty. He feigned madness but on interrogation Uko was able to convince the police that he was a fraudster.
The man was detained in the police custody while Uko was taken to the Government Children's home until he was proven innocent.
There was another scene when Uko was to be taken to the Children's home, the horse refused to leave him. Uko himself wept because he never wanted to miss the horse again. He suggested he should be alowed to stay in the zoo with the horse but was told he couldn't since he was not an animal.
By this time, the news had gone round the town that an old man who swindled a young boy had been caught and was in the police custody. Uko's father and the young men that were
assisting him to search for Uko were still in town when this incident happened. They got the news and ran quickly to the police station to rescue Uko.
However, there was a turn of event when the D.P.O (Departmental Police Officer) in charge of the station ordered that Mr. Ben and his men be detained. He directed that Uko should be brought to the station the following day for mnore interrogation.
After the investigation, it was proven that Uko was punished as a result of the old man's wickedness. His mother found it difficult to believe what he heard about his son. Can an old man do that to a little boy and why on earth would a father be so heartless to his own child to the point of sending him to the street for no cause?
She was dumbfounded and it was equally very difficult for her to follow the council members to the station. Women had always dreaded the Police Station. She really desired to see her son but wouldn't want to pass through the police to see him.
She dreaded men in uniform because of their guns. The council members were able to convince her to follow them to the station.
At the station, she was shocked to see her son in such a bad shape. She was touched beyond measures on seeing him. Uko too wept bitterly when he saw his mother. He couldn't narrate all he went through to his mother.
However, he told her how he was almost knocked down by a truck while selling water on the street. He also told her about Mrs. Sam who took care of him and how he raised money to start selling.
Uko was released to his mother after signing some documents with the Government officials. She was partially happy and partially ashamed because she was blamed for not reporting the incident to the police or the welfare office in her Community.
She went back to the village in company of some members of community as others were detained for failure to report the crime to the Police. She was saddened by the turn of event. If only her husband had heeded her advice this would have been

avoided.
Uko was happy to go back to the village with his mother but
he thought he would go back with his horse. He kept praying
that nothing bad would happen to it.
The Police had promised to release it to him as soon as the
case was over in court. He was told it will be used as an exhibit
in court against the fraudulent old man. He was consoled that
God who made him see the horse after many months of
torture will keep it safe until he reclaims it.
The moment the villagers caught sight of him they jubilant with songs and dances. He was
heralded as a hero, they were happy the son was proven innocent. There was jubilation
everywhere in the little town of Owie, the village square had become a Mecca of sort as
everybody tried to get a
picture of Uko.
On seeing his physique some wept while others poured curses on those who put him through
such pains. They also thanked God who kept him safe during the period of torture.
The news of Uko's home coming spread like wild fire in the neighbourhood and people were
trooping to the village square to catch sight of him. His grandmother who could not walk tried to
crawl to the place because she couldn't wait any longer to see her treasured grandson, Uko.
On sighting the poor woman crawling towards the village square, people told Uko who quickly ran
to meet her. "Grand ma", he cried raising her up as well. The old woman was short of words and
too shocked to talk, she only hugged her grand-son whom she had missed dearly.
Through the period he was away she rarely ate, played or went out. Many thought she wouldn't
survive the trauma of losing a boy who had always run errands for her. She refused to be
comforted. When one of her daughters who was married outside the village attempted to take her
so she could forget the
incident, she bluntly rejected the offer. She said it was better to die than live without the boy.
In fact, she was the only one who took Uko for his words. She embraced the tattered boy with
tears running down her cheeks and they were taken home on a motor cycle by a
relation.
On reaching home as he was removing the dirty clothes for a clean bath, Uko noticed the
controversial bean inside his pocket. It has been there since the day his father took him away, he
remembered he even tried to plant it behind the place thatharboured him in town.
To his dismay, it didn't grow over- night as the old man had promised. So he decided to keep it
convinced he had been jolted. Uko showed the bean to his mother who said it will also be used as
an exhibit against the man in court.
After the bath, Uko and the mother sat down to eat the meal prepared for them by their relations.
People had started bringing him gifts of all kinds. He had so lost his appetite that he couldn't eat,
this worried his mother greatly. She started crying again but she was consoled by the
sympathizers.
In the evening the whole village was thrown into uproar when it was realised that some members
of the village council were detained at the station. Wives started looking for their husbands and
children asked for their fathers. Some who had no food wept more since men were the bread
winners. It only dawned on them late as they were thinking the men may havebbeen enjoying
themselves in town.
They ought to have asked Uko's mother but were convinced they would come back on their own.
But what crime did they commit that would warrant their detention. Or was it wrong for them to
have gone there to defend Uko? They knew a little about the law, it was strange to hear that
refusing to report a crime committed in their community to the appropriate quarters was an
offence. They were only released two days after and it was the village head that went to bail them.
These men came back with their own story to tell about the police station and life behind the bars.
They regretted their
ignorance. The village head also promised to hire the services of a lawyer in handling cases in the
community. They learnt that ignorance to the law is no excuse.
After series of investigation, the old man and Mr. Ben were prosecuted. The executive members
of village pleaded for Ben's release but they were told the treatment he gave to Uko was not only

an offence against his child but a crime against the state.
They were told of the Child's Rights Law which had been signed and adopted by the state government. The old man was sentenced to six years imprisonment with hard labour for fraud and theft while Mr. Ben, Uko's father bagged three years
imprisonment for maltreating a minor.
The village head, chief Udo Ebong invited some officials of the Ministry of Women Affairs and Social Welfare to educate the parents on the Chld's Rights Law. The people were happy at the end of the session.
Mr. Akpan's family was saddened at the turn of event but was comforted that he will come back reformed since he had
been known for high handedness of his wives and children. He used to treat them like animals.
Uko's horse was handed back to him and he rode it back to the village with his mother after the ruling. Partially, he was happy and on the other, hand he was sad over his father's conviction.

HOW SHE CHANGED HER DRUNK HUSBAND

When a woman wants to teach you a lesson, even Satan sits down to take notes. My neighbour was a big drunk. His wife used to pick him up in bars and in trenches. Her family friends advised her to leave him but she was hopeful that she'll find a solution.

One Saturday she went to pick him again, he was completely drunk. Instead of taking him home, she headed straight to the mortuary. She negotiated with the mortuary attendants to make him lie with the corpses and when he wakes up, help me to teach him a lesson. She then went back home. Fear Women!

When he woke up, he started screaming when he found himself sleeping in the middle of dead bodies. He started screaming and calling for help pleading that he's not dead. The mortuary attendants came laughing and told him that they are used to corpses being brought to the morgue and start practice witchcraft. They told him to lie down and that he was dead and whatever he was seeing was not in real life but in the other end of living dead.

He continued screaming and the morgue attendants came with an axe and hammer and told him that stubborn corpses are beaten and hacked until they become cooperative. He was told to lie and wait for his postmortem later that day since his cause of death hadn't been established.

He stayed there frightened in the middle of corpses the whole of that day and Sunday night. On Monday morning they released him and told him to go home, say bye bye to his family and then come back to the morgue for preservation since he was now a mere spirit.

He ran home on foot, straight to the mirror to check if he was seeing himself. His wife pretended not to see him which made him even more worried. He went to the bathroom took a shower, dressed up and carried a Bible. That's when his wife told him that it was a Monday morning and not Sunday.
Several months later he's yet to reveal what happened to him and where he was the two nights he wasn't at home. He stopped taking alcohol completely, not even soda, just milk and water. He goes to church religiously.
The power of a woman!

THE UNGRATEFUL FOStER MOTHER

here lived a very rich woman with her only daughter in a city of Abaja. They could afford everything they needed in life but they were very stingy. The daughter was named Catherine but preferred to be called Catty. She was proud and rude, so people refused to associate with her One day, when she visited the village with her mother she
fell in love with Affiong who had just lost her parents.
Catherine pitied her and told her mother to bring the girl along to Abaja. She told her mum she really loved Affiong and would like to take her as a foster
sister since she was an only child.
Everybody was surprised including her mother because Catty has never shown such kindness to anyone even her relations. She was very
arrogant and snobby.
Catherine's mother visited Affiong's family where she met her extended family members. She told them her wish to adopt Affiong as her own
daughter since she has lost both parents. She promised to take good care of her and also sent her to school. She said she will attend the same school with Catty, her daughter.
The family thought it wise to give their consent. They felt there was no one else who could do that for her in the village.
They also considered the kind of exposure she would gain from living in the city and decided that Affiong should go with Catty.
Though her parents' burial wasn't yet fixed she was allowed to follow them as a consolation. Catty's mother had promised to assist in the burial arrangements. She also said she would attend the burial with Affiong whenever the date is fixed.
Affiong was very excited to leave the village for a better life in the city. She anticipated good fortune in her new family. She hadn't much to pack since her clothes were few. Affiong wasn't bothered because she would have more clothes from her new mother who has just given her some new set of clothes. So she only packed her few clothes into a cellophane bag. Off they set out to the city with joy while the villagers watched in bewilderment.
Other children envied her. They wished they could be given such opportunity. The children started discussing what it means to live in the city. Some said over there you don't need to work all you do is eat, watch television and play. They
dreamt of living there sometime when they have the opportunity.
Some of her friends were very delighted that their friend could find solace again in life. Affiong never really knew what joy looked like because she was denied of a good family bonding. She used to envy her friends who lived happily with
their parents.
Sometimes, she would pack her things to live with Abasifreke, her friend so that she could be happy but her mother would always go there to pick her. She was made to
believe that there was no place like home. How would she like her home when her parents were living like cats and dogs, they were always attacking each other.
Due to this kind of environment, she became very timid.
Among her friends, Affiong was the only one who lacked self esteem and confidence. They tried to build up her confidence but were hindered by her family background.
Since her parents were always barking at her, she would hardly expressed herself even when she was hurt. They knew
Affiong will be missed in school but she had no option than to leave her problems behind to pursue a brighter future. She was a kind and loving girl.
Affiong wasn't only living with the Ozi's as one of their own but was adopted by them as promised. She was to have equal right as Catty, her sister.
Before her adoption, she bore Affiong John Pius but she had to change to Favour Paul Ozi. She was registered in Catty's school but was in a lower class. Though they were of the same age, her

academic ability was low considering where
she came from.

Catherine opted to teach her how to read and write. She also taught her how to eat with cutlery and speak good English so that she would be able to fit in well in her new community. Her mother bought more shoes and clothes for her. She was also given a box for her clothes and she could hardly believe life could be that fair to her.

She was very fast at learning but was a bit timid in holding the cutlery. She chose to eat with hand or spoon as she wasn't very comfortable with the English ways. Even her teachers commended her for adjusting fast but she was having some difficulty in areas like Mathematics. Vouho Composition and Industrial Arts.

These inefficiencies affected her scores in the Terminal Exams but in the Promotion Exams she did excellently well even better than Catty who was always on the average. Their mother decided to reward Affiong's good performance in school by buying her a toy laptop. However, she didn't buy anything for Catty. Catty became very bitter and unhappy.

Catty was very jealous of Afiong, she felt aggrieved and would rarely talk to her unlike before. Initially, Affiong did not notice her change in behaviour but was forced to confront her when she started to notice Catty wasn't happy with her.

Unfortunately, this provoked Catty more than she would have expected, she flared up and started raining abuses on her. Affiong was surprised at her reaction but had no right again to complain. When their mother returned in the

evening, Catty told her a cooked story. She said Affiong has been abusing her ever since she passed her exams. She also said that Affiong has been calling her silly names. Mrs. Ovi was infuriated and vowed to deal with Affiong for abusing her only child. Henceforth, certain rights and privileges were withdrawn from her. She was to be treated as a maid and an orphan that she was.

Meanwhile, Affiong regretted having followed them as they were making life miserable for her. She had no right to watch the Television, not even in the evenings when everybody was gathered around it. She only ate alone in the kitchen.

Sometimes, she ate the crumbs of what others ate. Their dog had more privileges than she did. All her expectations of finding solace were once again dashed. Indeed, she was
dejected and wished to go back to the village.

The worst happened when she was withdrawn from school for no sincere reasons. She was told the school could not accommodate her due to her poor performance in Yoruba but Affiong knew it was a lie. Catty has always hated competition, so wouldn't live to see
a maid overtake her academically and socially. Why should her own mother buy gifts for a maid without giving her anything?

Affiong was deceived she could do better in trade since she wasn't good academically. She was also told school was not for her type. She became timid again, making more mistakes than ever and this attracted her foster mother's anger. Her new job was to do home chores. She would mop the whole house,   wash dishes and do laundry for Catty.

The house help was asked to do a few things like cooking for the family and going to the market so that Affiong would not be idle. She too wasn't kind to her as she had always envied her position as an adopted child. All these happened after the funeral of her parents. If it had happened earlier, she wouldnt
have come back with them city.

She longed to go back to her village where everybody lived as a community, sharing things in common. Anytime she remembered the free, fair and compulsory education implemented in her state from Primary to Secondary schools
she would weep her eyes out.

If she were in the village, she would have gone to school and her grandmother would have catered for her in the absence of her parents. Her uncle used to buy text books and exercise books for her when her parents were alive. They
would have still been there for her.

Affiong remembered with nostalgia how she used to play with her friends in the village. She was the favourite of her friends. In the village, she used to play on her way to the stream. They would play around their house at night after

dinner especially during the new moon. She could eat with her
cousins anytime she was hungry. After each meal, the fish and
periwinkle would be shared among those who ate the food.
They did not have sumptuous meals to eat on well decorated tables but they were very happy and
contented with what they had. They had no luxury   but were very happy to share all they had
together.
She wished her friends and relations in the village would
begin to value our community life. Those in the village longed to go to the city believing that the
best is found there. Little do they know that many children who are taken to towns by relations
are treated like dogs.
This thought made her homesick and she couldn't hide her feelings any longer, so, she wept until
her foster mother and Catty returned. Mrs. Ovi met her crying and never cared to ask what was
wrong.
She only shouted at her when she discovered she hasn't washed the dishes. She snarled at her as
usual but Affiong refused to budge. She told her boldly she would like to go back to her grand-
parents.
This provoked the Ovis who descended on her like a goat.
She was given the beating of her life for insulting madam.
That night the poor girl went to bed without food. She was completely disorganised.
Earlier, when there was a good relationship between Catty and Affiong they had shared their
families' secrets. Affiong told her disgustful things about her parents.
She disclosed everything both true and false about her parents to Catty. She said that her parents
were a very young couple who gave birth to her out of wedlock.. She narrated how her father used
to fight her mother regularly. "One day, my parents were having an argument and my father
rushed to his room, brought out his machete and wanted to slaughter my mother. She screamed
at the top of her voice. Thank goodness this attracted our relatives who ran o.
to rescue her. If not he would have killed my mother in cold blood", she narrated. Oh, can a
husband do that to her wife? I can't imagine that. My
father has been kind to my mum. They are two loved birds who could not harm each other", Caty
exclaimed.
Every evening, the two sisters would sit together to discuss what happened in their school.
Affiong told her how her parents died in a ghastly motor accident. Catty rendered her sincere
condolences and wiped her tears as she started
sobbing remembering what she suffered as a child. Catty consoled her. Definitely, she was
consoled and she never wept again until the turnof event.
She tried to figure out what she did to annoy Catty and that whole family but could I not point out
any. She then decided to apologise to her at night when she must have retired to bed They used
to share the same room but since her quarrel with Catty, she wasn't allowed there again but was
given a place to keep her things at the lobby behind the dinning. She
attempted to meet Catty but she refused to let her inn.
Life became so unbearable for her that she almost ran away. She had thought of confiding in her
Sunday school teacher but couldn't reach her since she was no longer allowed to go to church
even on Sundays. That was luxury to her, so she was asked to stay back to clean the house every
Sunday.
One day, after the whole family had gone out she dared to switch on the television for the first
time. Incidentally, there was a Programme on Child Labour and Trafficking of persons, this
attracted her attention and she paid attention to it.
At the end of the talk, some telephone numbers were given to the public for complaint and
distress calls. She called one of
the numbers with the house phone and the receiver happened to be the Director of National
Agency for The Prohibition in Trafficking of Persons {NAPTIP}.
She narrated her ordeal to the man and told him never to call the line so that her mother would
not know she called them. She was asked to give the details of her foster mother and was told
not to run away in order not to miss out. She was
also assured she would be rescued immediately.
The following morning being a Monday, officials of NAPTIP visited their house and rescued her as

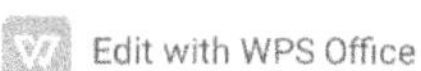

promised. Mrs. Ovi was arrested though she pleaded to be given time to report at the station with her lawyer. At the station she was asked to make statement on the allegations of child labour and molestation of a minor Affiong was taken to the Ministry of Women Affairs and Social Welfare for registration. Later she was taken to Government Children's home and she had a good time there with other children.

There, she had equal rights and attended one of the best schools in town. The news got to the village and people were afraid to give their children to ive with rich people in cities.

The Ovis shocked the whole village, nobody would believe they could treat an orphan like that. Catty regretted her actions and wished they could be retracted but it was a little late as her mother would have to pay dearly for her actions. She was sent to jail for the abuse done to a minor though, she tried to avert justice by bribing the lawyers. Her money couldn't help her avert justice.

Her husband had to fly in from France to witness the ruling and to hire the best lawyers for her. However, when he got home to know the kind of maltreatment meted on the poor little girl he was shocked.

When he read from his daughter's confessional statement he was afraid to meddle into such affairs. He told the officials handling the case that he had always advised his family not to be inhumane. He said he had to employ the services of a mature person asa maid to avoid hiring children.

He disclosed that his wife hasn't been very nice to others which informed the need to employ adults as her maid. Mr. Ovi had to go back to France with his only daughter so she could be well groomed. He saw the need to teach her how to treat others like human beings.

Before Catty left with her father she asked to meet Affiong, so she could ask for forgiveness. Her father took her to the government children's home where he also apologised on
behalf of the family. He offered to pay her for the damage done to the poor girl.

He wanted to take her along but could not since she was maltreated by the same family. Mr. Ovi was told that the state government would take good care of Affiong, so he didn't need to pay her for the harm done by his wife.

Affiong was happy to reconcile with her friend, Catty who asked for forgiveness. She confessed she had long forgiven them and would always be grateful to the family for the favour she received during the period she lived with them. She also asked the officials to pardon her foster mother so that she could be free again but this couldn't be granted since the offence wasn't only committed against her, it was an offence against the state and humanity.

However, Mrs. Ovi was only given a year jail term since she pl 猫 aded guilty. Affiong promised she would always be there for her and refused to change her name to foster her relationship with the family.

She also promised to go back to the family when she comesof age. The little orphan was happy to be free again. She was equally glad to live among other children who were nice to her.

There she had equal rights as other children. The officials were quite nice. The children in the home were
considered government children. The governor was their father and the wife of the governor was their mother while the Commissioner for Women Affairs and Social Welfare was their second mother. She visited them regularly to ensure they were properly taken care of.

END

THE KING'S   DAUGHTER

Once upon a time, there lived a rich and prosperous king, named King Alade. King Alade was the ruler of a very large kingdom, he was a king who was loved by his subjects
because he was wise, kind and most importantly, he was not a tyrant.
The Kingdom prospered under his rule, there was no famine and plenty of food was in is circulation. He did not tax his people more
than they could bear, his soldiers protected the kingdom from invaders and the King was a
wise judge who settled matters amicably amongst his people.
The people were happy because they had a great king who listened to their needs and they loved him very much. But, as great as King Alade was, he had one problem, he had no Sons.
King Alade had seven children in total and all of them were girls. His seven daughters, Adeola, Damilola, Funmi, Tinu, Wunmi, Folake and Wonu. All of his daughters were intelligent, smart
and beautiful and very hardworking. The King really loved and cherished his daughters dearly, he wanted the best for them and had even been thinking of making his first
daughter, Adeola the heir to his throne. But, there was a problem.
The King had an evil Prime Minister who secretly wanted to become the King, he wanted to take over the Kingdom and make the people suffer, so he began to whisper evil
thoughts into the King's head.
"Your majesty, people will think you are a weak King if you let Adeola become your heir." The Prime Minister told the King, "But why?" The King asked. "Adeola is intelligent, she is smart, she is beautiful, she is a great warrior, better than most warriors in my Kingdom and she is capable of making good decisions. I think people as their would be happy to have her ruler after I join my fathers." The King countered. "Yes it is true, Adeola is all of that but she is a girl. It is not something that is done. A woman cannot rule over the Kingdom, the people would hate you. They would curse you after your death that you let them be ruled by a Woman.
King Alade pondered over his Prime
Minister's words. It is true that a woman has never led the kingdom but what could he do when he was blessed with only girls. All his
children were qualified enough to rule but Adeola was the most qualified.
"So what do you suggest I do, Prime
Minister?" King Alade asked. The Prime Minister smiled, that was exactly the question he wanted the King to ask him because he had a plan, a very evil plan. "Your Majesty, It would be better to marry husband proves worthy, he would become the King after you." The Prime Minister suggested. "Are you sure this would work, I don't think I trust anyone apart from Adeola to rule the Kingdom after me. Besides, Adeola doesn't have many suitors." The King said doubtfully that the Prime Minister's plan would work.
"Your Majesty, organise a contest. Bring all the greatest warriors in the Kingdom together and let them contest for the hand of Princess Adeola. Let the best nan win.," The Prime Minister suggested.
The King thought about and agreed that it was a good idea, he knew his daughter well, she would not want to marry a man who wasn't strong or wise so it would be better to hold a contest but he also knew that he had to discuss the matter with his He summoned his daughter, Princess Adeola and told her of the plan that he and the Prime Minister had come up with. "Father, this is so sudden. Why do you want me to marry all of a sudden?" Princess Adeola asked her father.
"I want you to rule after me when I die but the Prime Minister told me that the Kingdom would not accept you as their ruler. That it would be better if your husband ruled instead." The King explained.
Princess Adeola listened intensely to her father's explanation but the truth was that she did not

trust the Prime Minister. But because her father was very sad and she wanted to make him happy she agreed to the marriage Contest. Princess Adeola greatly distrusted the Prime Minister, he was acting sneaky so she suspected that he had other plans for her. So, she told her six sisters of their father's plan and told them to be watchful of the Prime Minister, because he seemed to have plans of his own.

Truthfully, the Prime Minister had other plans. On the day of the contest, warriors came from all over the Kingdom to fight for the hand of the princess. The day of the contest was a very joyful day, there were

dancers and drummers from the cultural troupe who entertained the guests before the contest began.

The Prime Minister had organised for some hood lumns to kidnap the Princess while everywhere was rowdy. When it was time for the contest to begin, Princess Adeola had been kidnapped.

The entire Kingdom was thrown into a frenzy, who could have done such a thing? They all cried and wailed, their favourite princess had been kidnapped. But the six sisters knew who to suspect, their sister had warned them beforehand to be wary of the Prime Minister. King Alade's fragile old heart could not take the sudden disappearance of his beloved daughter, he hurt so much that he died from the pain of losing his daughter. And since he

did not name an heir before he died the Kingdom automatically fell to the Prime Minister and so the evil Prime Minister became the King,

The new King laughed evilly to himself, his plan had worked, the king had died due to the disappearance of his daughter and now he was king. Now it was time to rule. He was a bad King, he taxed the people heavily, he cheated them out of their birthright, he was wicked and irresponsible and a tyrant and soon the once prosperous Kingdom became a shadow of its self and the people suffered greatly. The remaining six sisters could no longer stand the evil reign of the Prime Minister, they could not stand the suffering of the people.

The Prime Minister had not been King for long but the Kingdom was already in a terrible state.

They could not let him continue to reign, they had to do something about it, they were all warriors but they needed the right heir to be

on the throne. So, Damilola the second eldest sister after Adeola gathered her sisters for secret meeting because the new King had

forbidden them from seeing each other because he knew the sisters were very close to each other and he knew if they were together they would be a force fo reckon with.

"My sisters, " Damilola began, "We cannot continue to watch the usurper take control of the Kingdom. We must do something about this, the people are suffering." She continued. "It is true, my sister but what can We do, the people are too broken to rise up and fight against the tyrannical ruler," Wunmi said. "Not if we find the rightful heir to the throne." Folake said. Her sisters perked up at this statement.

"We all know that our father wanted Adeola to rule but the evil Prime Minister convinced him to do otherwise and organise that stupid

contest,"Folake backed up her statement and her sisters nodded in agreement. "We have to find our sister, she is a great warrior and she can turn this thing arOund," Tinu said. "The question now is, how do we find her?" Wonu asked.

"Our father raised us better than this, he didn't raise us to always doubt ourselves, he raised us as warriors, as intelligent women, as

skilled huntsmen and we would do his memory a disservice if we give up now," Damilola said. We would journey to the end of the world if We have to but we must find our sister and Bring her back home with us. She is the rightful heir to the throne, she will bring an end to this tyranny." Wonu said, suddenly motivated by her sister's speech. And so, the sisters set themselves on ajourney

to find their sister, it was a tedious journey because they had no clue where Adeola had been taken to but they had to try. For so many reasons, they could not fail their mission.

They loved their sister and missed her greatly and they also needed her back home so that all that was wrong could be righted. The sisters crossed seven rivers and seven

seas, they climbed seven mountains, they were guided by their goodwill and intentions.

They finally found their sister, Adeola, she had been sold into slavery to a far far away kingdom. The sisters were shocked to find thief sister. a great warrior chained down like a dog and made to all sort of jobs that, no one should be made to do. They approached their sister cautiously, they did not want to attract the slave masters. Immediately Adeola saw her sisters she recognised them.

A sudden gladness came over her heart she had been waiting for her sisters for a long time, they were strong warriors they would help free her and the rest ofthe slaves.

"Welcome my sisters, I have been waiting for you for a long time. I am glad that you have finally found me." She whispered. "How did this happen? How can a great princess and the heir to a great Kingdom be

trapped like this?" Damilola asked, her eyes were red with anger.

"Keep your voice down, we don't want to attract the slave masters ," Wonu whispered. it is the evil Prime Minister who organised for some hoodlums to kidnap me and bring

me here. They attacked me from the back and disarmed me before I could attack them. That's why I am here."Adeola explained.

"How is father doing?" She asked. Her sisters became really sad and tears filled their eyes as they told Adeola that the King had passed

away due to grief.

Adeola cried with her sisters, she had loved her father so much and now she would never see him again because of the evil Prime Minister. They had to teach the Prime

Minister a lesson that he would not forget in a lifetime. The sisters quickly set up a plan to free Adeola

and the other slaves. They pretended to be slaves caught by the slave masters, they hid their weapons under their clothes and when the slave masters locked them up with the other slaves. They freed the slaves and their sister with the weapons they had Snuck into the slave camp. They fought the: slave masters and won the battle attract the slave masters ," Wonu whispered. it is the evil Prime Minister who organised for some hoodlums to kidnap me and bring

me here. They attacked me from the back and disarmed me before I could attack them. That's why I am here."Adeola explained.

"How is father doing?" She asked. Her sisters became really sad and tears filled their eyes as they told Adeola that the King had passed

away due to grief.

Adeola cried with her sisters, she had loved her father so much and now she would never see him again because of the evil Prime Minister. They had to teach the Prime

Minister a lesson that he would not forget in a lifetime. The sisters quickly set up a plan to free Adeola

and the other slaves. They pretended to be slaves caught by the slave masters, they hid their weapons under their clothes and when the slave masters locked them up with the other slaves. They freed the slaves and theire the slaves were now tree to most of them decided to stay with go but Adeola and her six sisters to follow them back to their Kingdom and help them win the battle against the evil Prime Minister.

Adeola was moved by the loyalty of the former slaves and she accepted to take them back with her to her Kingdom. They journeyed back their Kingdom, they had to Cross the seven rivers, seven seas and seven:

mountains to get back to their Kingdom but this time the journey was easier because they bad accomplished their mission and they had joy and hope in their hearts that they could defeat the evil King. When they returned to the Kingdom, the people were so happy to see Adeola, they carried her high on their shoulders. They were

happy that their rightful ruler was back and would defeat the Prime Minister and bring peace and happiness back to the Kingdom. One of the evil King's spies quickly ran to the Palace to tell him that Princess Adeola and her sisters had returned to the Kingdom and they were being celebrated by the people. "Impossible!" He yelled.

"She cannot be back, I made sure she disappeared for good. How did she get back into my Kingdom?" He asked, he was yelling, his eyes were red with anger but also with fear. He knew that now that the rightful heir to the throne had returned nobody would listen to him anymore. He had to get rid of her again. "You! You! You!" He yelled at three of his

guards, go and gather the other guards, we must fight that fake princess. "She thinks she can come back into this kingdom and take

what is mine. I will show her who the real ruler is." He added. He fidgeted and began to place

about his chambers frantic and unsure of what to do. "Did you not hear me?" He yelled at the guards when they did not make a move to follow his orders. The rightful heir was back and everybody including his guards were tired of his tyranny.
"Fine, if you will not do it, I will go out and fight her for myself." He yelled and went outside to fight the Princess but he was met with a very angry crowd carrying the Princess
high on their shoulders. They were happy with her but angry with him.
"How dare you?! I am the King here not this ordinary woman." He yelled.
"We know what you did, you lied to our King that we would not accept our Princess as our ruler because she is woman and that is not true we don't care about her being a woman, she is kind, wise and just and she would protect us because she is a true ruler like her father, a worthy Queen." One of the subjects said to the evil Prime Minister turned King. "You don't know what you are talking about, she left you, she ran away because she did not want to be King, she hates all of you." The Prime Minister lied. that's a lie, you bad her kidnapped and Sold unto slavery. it was that grief of losing her that led to her father's death. You are a kidnapper, a liar and a murderer. And we don't want you, we are grateful to the Princesses for bringing
back our rightful heir. Who knows what would have happened under your reign?" Another subject said.
"That's enough everyone. I have made my decision. This evil King does not deserve to leave among us. So, for his crimes against us, I am sending him into exile." Queen Adeola decreed and everybody gave a shout of joy. Their Queen was a good leader, she could have had him executed but out of the goodness of her heart, she sent him on exile Instead. Although fate and karma had different plans for the evil King, he died on a lonely road with no one beside him, no wealth, no title. His greed led him to his death while Queen Adeola, her six Sisters and the rest of the Kingdom prospered and lived happily ever after.

THE END